High Blood Pressure

How to Lower Blood Pressure Naturally and Prevent Heart Disease

Christina Neal

The trademarks that are used are without any consent, and the publication of the trademark is without permission or backing by the trademark owner. All trademarks and brands within this book are for clarifying purposes only and are owned by the owners themselves, not affiliated with this document.

Table of Contents

Introduction

Currently, 75 million people suffer from hypertension in the United States. Hypertension was responsible for 410,000 deaths in 2014. Although family history and aging can increase your chance of having hypertension, an unhealthy lifestyle remains the primary cause. Lack of exercise, eating junk food, not drinking enough water, or lack of sleep can all lead to an elevated blood pressure.

Most drugs on the market target the symptoms of high blood pressure and are not designed to address the actual source of hypertension. Medicines alone aren't enough to treat your problem in the long run.

With this book, you will develop a comprehensive understanding of hypertension and its ill effects so you can take the required preventive measures to keep it from getting worse. This book focuses on the symptoms, causes, and treatment options for hypertension, and the various complications that can result. It will help you learn more about beneficial lifestyle changes, the DASH diet plan, and herbal supplements and medications that will allow you to take control of your health and start lowering your blood pressure for good.

High blood pressure does not control your life. There are lifestyle changes you can make to regain control. If you don't know where to start, this book will guide you through your journey. Get ready to find some long-term solutions to your blood pressure problems.

Happy reading!

Chapter 1: What is High Blood Pressure

Our hearts pump life-giving blood to our organs via arteries. Blood pressure is the force by which blood is pushed through the arteries. High blood pressure is a condition where your blood pressure levels drastically increase.

High blood pressure is a "silent killer," because it often shows no obvious symptoms for a long time. It is estimated that 33% of those that have high blood pressure are not even aware they have the disease. However, hypertension cannot be taken lightly. If left untreated, hypertension will cause serious damage to the heart and overall health.

There are two main types of hypertension: when the cause of high blood pressure is unknown, it's called essential hypertension; when the cause of high blood pressure is the result of a known condition or disease, it's called secondary hypertension. An estimated 90% of hypertension cases are essential hypertension. By contrast, secondary hypertension is sudden and blood pressure levels are much higher than in essential hypertension.

Understanding Blood Pressure Readings

Blood pressure rises as the heart beats or contracts. This is referred to as systolic pressure. It falls between heartbeats, which is known as diastolic pressure.

Your blood pressure rises and falls throughout the day. If you are asleep, your blood pressure will be lower than when you are awake. A typical daily range includes 10-15 millimeters of mercury (mmHg) on the systolic pressure and 5-10 mmHg on the diastolic pressure. Other factors also affect your blood pressure, such as mood and physical activities.

When you go for a blood pressure check-up, the nurse inflates a cuff on your arm with air and measures your blood pressure with a blood pressure monitor. The blood pressure reading is given as a ratio, for example, 120/80. This is read as 120 over 80. The first—or top—number is your systolic pressure (120 mmHg), and the lower number is the diastolic pressure (90 mmHg). The systolic number measures pressure in the arteries as the heart beats and pumps blood. The diastolic number measures the pressure in between heartbeats, as the blood returns to the heart.

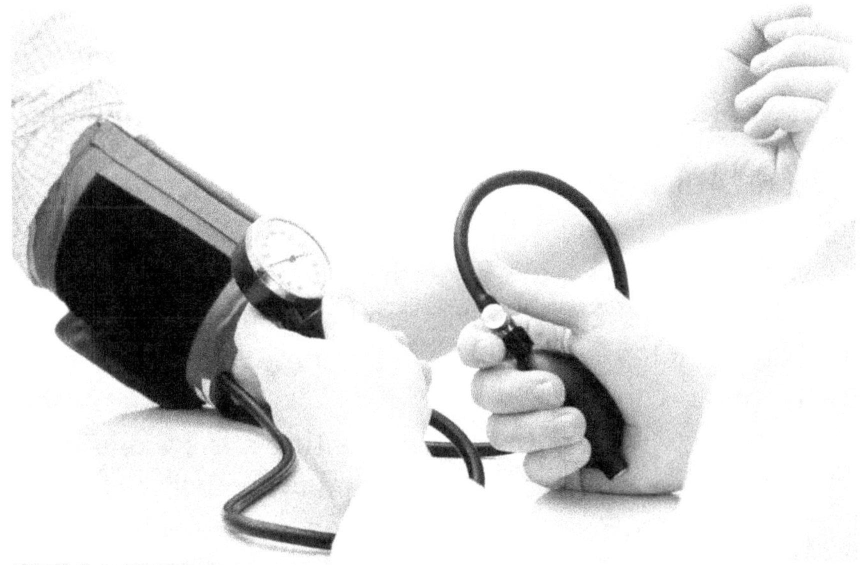

The normal blood pressure level is below 120/80. When your reading is between 120/80 and 139/89, you are pre-hypertensive—meaning you are at a higher risk for high blood pressure. A reading above 140/90 is considered high blood pressure.

When your doctor notices your blood pressure reading is higher than 120/80, he or she may suggest you monitor blood pressure at home over a period of time to make sure the elevated blood pressure is not caused by temporary factors. If your blood pressure is 140/90 or higher and remains at that level during the observation period, you will be diagnosed with high blood pressure. If you have a chronic disease, such as diabetes or kidney disease, a constant blood pressure reading of 130/80 or higher is considered high blood pressure.

You will need to regularly monitor your blood pressure moving forward. It is easy to measure and track your blood pressure at home using a blood pressure meter. There are digital versions if you do not know how to use a conventional sphygmomanometer.

What causes high blood pressure?

The exact cause of hypertension remains unknown in 90% of hypertension cases (essential hypertension). Research has shown there are several risk factors associated with high blood pressure. When these factors are present, a person is at a higher risk of developing the disease.

Aging–As we age, the risk of hypertension increases. Men are more likely to develop high blood pressure in their middle ages, at around 45 years old. Women more often develop the disease in their 60s.

As we age, what often happens is that our systolic blood pressure becomes higher and the diastolic number lower. This is called isolated systolic hypertension and effects 60% of people with high blood pressure. Aging makes our arteries narrower and stiffer and our hearts just a little less efficient than they used to be.

Ethnicity–Serious complications from high blood pressure are more common in African Americans. It has been observed that, on average, African Americans develop the disease at a younger age than Caucasians.

Family History–High blood pressure tends to run in families. If your parents have it, it is wise to avoid risk factors to lower your chances of developing the disease.

Obesity–When you are overweight, you need more blood to supply the organs with oxygen and nutrients. Since more blood is needed, the heart pumps harder and blood pressure increases. People who are obese are twice as likely to develop high blood pressure, since they are also more susceptible to secondary hypertension due to high cholesterol.

Smoking–Every time you smoke a cigarette, your blood pressure rises, but the greatest damage caused by smoking is to the arteries. Over time, the chemicals present in cigarettes can cause your arteries to narrow, thus increasing the pressure necessary to pump blood throughout the body.

Lack of Physical Activity–A sedentary lifestyle often leads to being overweight, which increases the risk of having elevated blood pressure levels.

Stress–While there is no proof that stress causes long-term hypertension, it certainly temporarily raises your blood pressure. It is the activities associated with stress, such as smoking, overeating, and lack of sleep, that eventually cause hypertension. The hormones produced by your body when you're stressed can also damage the arteries and increase blood pressure.

Too Much Alcohol–If you drink more than three glasses in one sitting, it will temporarily raise your blood pressure levels. If you are a binge drinker, alcohol will eventually lead to hypertension. Alcohol contains calories that will make you gain unwanted weight.

Lack of Vitamin D–Research has linked low vitamin D levels with cases of high blood pressure, however, research has yet to prove if vitamin D supplements can lower blood pressure levels in people who are already hypertensive.

Too Much Sodium Intake–A diet high in salt disrupts the body's sodium balance and causes water retention. The increased amount of fluids raises blood pressure.

Lack of Potassium–Potassium counters the blood pressure effects of sodium. If you have a salt-heavy diet and you don't meet the recommended 4,700 mg potassium daily intake, the chances of having high blood pressure may increase.

Kidney Disease–The majority of people with kidney disease have high blood pressure. This is called renal hypertension, which is caused by a narrowing of the arteries that deliver blood to the kidneys. When it doesn't get enough blood flow, the kidney reacts by acting as if it's dehydrated, releasing hormones that make the body retain sodium and water. The blood vessels fill with extra fluids and the result is high blood pressure.

Drug Use–Some drugs cause secondary hypertension. These include amphetamines, ecstasy, cocaine, corticosteroids, estrogens and other hormones, OTC coughs, colds and asthma medications, migraine medications, and nasal decongestants.

What are the symptoms of hypertension?

If you have high blood pressure, you might notice the following signs: dizziness, shortness of breath, chest pains, blurry vision, confusion, severe headache, or extreme fatigue.

It is important that you check your blood pressure before feeling these symptoms, because by the time you feel the symptoms, your blood pressure levels might be flying off the charts. If your blood pressure is in the pre-hypertensive range (120/80 – 139/89) or higher, you should have your blood pressure checked every year.

Emergency hypertension symptoms

When emergency hypertension signs occur, they may require immediate attention and need to be treated as a medical emergency. This condition is known as hypertensive crisis. A hypertensive crisis occurs when your blood pressure count reads beyond 180 for systolic pressure, or it goes beyond 110 for diastolic pressure. If you happen to check your own blood pressure using a monitor and notice a reading that high, do not panic. Wait for some time before taking another reading to make sure it's correct. If you get the same reading again, contact your physician immediately to set up an appointment. You can also call 911 emergency services to get you to an emergency room without wasting any more time. Some of the other signs of hypertensive crisis are:

- severe headaches,
- extreme anxiety,
- nose bleeds, and
- shortness of breath.

Emergency hypertensive crisis can result in life-threatening complications, such as stroke and heart attack.

Chapter 2: Hypertension Complications

Hypertension can cause the quiet deterioration of your body over the years, though it may take a long time for the symptoms to show. Uncontrolled hypertension can cause complications that are life-threatening. If you suffer from hypertension, it's imperative you visit your doctor for routine checkups. Below are some of the most common complications experienced by high blood pressure patients.

Cardiovascular Diseases

The high pressure being exerted on artery walls can damage blood vessels and the heart over time, causing cardiovascular disease.

- **Stroke**–Hypertension may lead to the damaging and narrowing of the arteries that supply the brain. In the worst case scenarios, the arteries are cut-off, leading to stroke. In fact, two-thirds of those who suffer their first stroke have elevated blood pressure.
- **Heart Failure**–High blood pressure causes the heart to work harder in order to pump blood through the body. The heart muscles thicken and weakens in time, and the heart may not be able to pump properly, resulting in heart failure.
- **Hypertensive Heart Disease**–The left ventricle becomes enlarged and the cardiac output decreases. When left untreated, this can lead to heart failure.
- **Arrhythmia**–High blood pressure can lead to disturbances in the heart's electrical signals, causing heartbeat irregularities.
- **Aneurysm**–This is when the walls of the arteries weaken and burst, which causes internal bleeding.

Diabetes

Diabetes and hypertension have a strong connection. High blood pressure can worsen diabetes complications, such as nephropathy and retinopathy. People with diabetes need to keep their blood pressure at 130/80 mmHg or lower in order to prevent further complications.

Kidney Disease

An estimated 30% of all cases of end-stage renal disease or kidney failure are caused by high blood pressure. Those who have been diagnosed with both diabetes and hypertension should closely watch the condition of their kidneys.

Dementia (Memory Loss)

Uncontrolled high blood pressure can lead to a diminished capacity to think, learn, and remember.

Loss of Vision

High blood pressure can also affect a person's vision. The blood vessels in the eyes can be torn, narrowed, or thickened, causing vision problems.

Sexual Dysfunction

Men who have high blood pressure may develop erectile dysfunction. It was previously thought that the drugs used for hypertension treatment caused the erection problems, but evidence now suggests that hypertension itself is the cause.

Chapter 3: Medicines and Supplements for High Blood Pressure

If you are diagnosed with high blood pressure, your doctor will prescribe medication to keep your blood pressure level normal. The following are medicines commonly prescribed. They are either meant to dilate the arteries or reduce water content in the blood to lower blood pressure and the heart's workload.

Medications for High Blood Pressure

Diuretics–are used to help the kidneys eliminate sodium and water in the body, thus reducing blood volume.

Angiotensin-Converting Enzyme (ACE) Inhibitors–help relax blood vessels by inhibiting the formation of a group of specific molecules that retain salt and water in the body and make the blood vessels constrict.

Angiotensin II Receptor Blockers (ARB)–also help relax blood vessels by stopping the action of the group of molecules that retain salt and water in the body and narrow the vessels.

Beta Blockers–reduce the heart's workload by dilating the blood vessels. The result is that the heart doesn't need to beat as fast to supply the body with blood.

Calcium Channel Blockers (CCB)–inhibit the movement of calcium into muscle cells in the heart and arterial walls, which widens the arteries and lowers blood pressure.

Vasodilators–open the blood vessels by relaxing muscle cells in arterial walls.

Long-term use of some of these medications may have harmful side effects. If you are taking hypertension medication, it is important to visit your doctor for an annual physical exam.

Herbal Medicines

Herbal medicines have been used to treat illness for ages. Some herbs have been studied and reported to have anti-hypertensive properties.

Garlic–has been studied extensively for its various health benefits. Allicin, the sulfur-containing compound in garlic, can lower blood pressure and protect the heart. Studies have shown that patients who were given garlic tablets for a period of two months had decreased blood pressure levels.

Celery–is a popular treatment for high blood pressure in China. Celery juice is mixed with honey and 8 ounces of the mixture is taken three times a day for one week. Compounds in celery relax muscle cells in arterial walls which explains its effectiveness in lowering blood pressure.

Hawthorn Berry–offers heart health benefits, including the prevention of clots, reduced blood pressure, and improved blood circulation. It can be taken as tea.

Cat's Claw–is used to treat hypertension and neurological problems, too! It reduces blood pressure by working on the calcium channels in muscle cells. It can be taken in supplement form and is available in most health stores.

Motherwort–is an herb belonging to the mint family. It contains a compound called leonurine which promotes the relaxation of arterial walls. It also contains antioxidants which also reduce blood pressure. Motherwort is available in health stores as a supplement.

Vitamin and Mineral Supplements

You don't need to take vitamin supplements if you're already eating a well-balanced diet, such as the DASH diet. However, if you feel you aren't getting enough vitamins and minerals in your diet, here's a list of supplements that can help maintain normal blood pressure.

Vitamin D–If you're deficient in vitamin D, you are more prone to hypertension. Studies have shown that vitamin D supplements can lower the risk of high blood pressure. Unlike other nutrients, vitamin D is produced by our bodies when we are exposed to sunlight. If you are getting at least 20 minutes of sun exposure a day and eating a balanced diet, you probably don't need vitamin D supplements.

Vitamin C–Vitamin C has been shown to relax blood vessels and lower blood pressure. Natural sources of vitamin C include yellow bell pepper, guava, oranges, and Brussels sprouts, to name a few.

Vitamin E–Vitamin E has been proven to lower blood pressure in those with mild high blood pressure and reduce the risk of heart disease. You can find this antioxidant in foods such as pumpkin, tofu, spinach, sunflower seeds, avocado, and broccoli.

Magnesium–This mineral is closely linked to blood pressure. The recommended dosage of magnesium per day is 320 mg for adult women and 420 mg for adult men. Magnesium can be found in spinach, kale, soybeans, nuts and seeds, and salmon.

Coenzyme Q10–Some people with hypertension are deficient in CoQ10 which is also known as ubiquinone. Studies have shown that a daily dose of 45 to 60 mg CoQ10 can lower blood pressure by up to 25 mmHg. CoQ10 is an essential molecule produced by our bodies which our cells use to produce energy. Natural sources of CoQ10 include salmon, tuna, beef, chicken, peanuts, and broccoli.

Potassium–This mineral works by reducing the amount of fluids in the body and countering the effects of sodium on blood pressure. Potassium can be found in green vegetables such as spinach and kale, bananas, orange juice, white beans, sweet potatoes, and more.

Herbal medicines and dietary supplements are alternative treatments to battling high blood pressure. Before taking herbs and supplements with your prescribed medications, consult your doctor to make sure the combined effects are not excessive.

Chapter 4: Healthy Lifestyles to Lower Blood Pressure

Healthy lifestyles and natural remedies can help you lower blood pressure naturally. These alternative treatments will enable you to eradicate risk factors for hypertension and maybe even lower the dosage of your medication. This lifestyle of which we speak includes habits that should be followed by anyone wanting to live a healthy life.

Keep a Track of Your Blood Pressure Levels at Home

It's about time you get yourself a blood pressure monitoring device to help you keep tabs on your blood pressure on a regular basis. This device can alert you large fluctuations in your blood pressure levels. There is a wide range of blood pressure monitors available online and in stores. Ask your doctor for suggestions as to which model you should purchase.

Getting a blood pressure tracking device doesn't mean skipping regular doctor's visits. When your blood pressure is under control, you might not have to visit your doctor as often. However, if your blood pressure levels remain high, talk to your doctor immediately.

Watch Your Weight

Studies have shown that weight loss can lower the risk of high blood pressure by 28-40%. In addition, weight loss lowers the risks of other illnesses, such as type 2 diabetes, high cholesterol, and heart disease. If you are overweight, losing 5–10% of your body weight can significantly reduce your high blood pressure.

A good way to determine if you are overweight is by checking your body mass index (BMI) which measures your weight against your height. A BMI between 25 and 30 is considered overweight; 30 or more is obese. You can track your BMI using an online BMI calculator. For those with high blood pressure, a BMI of 25 or less is ideal.

The simplest way to lose weight is by eating fewer calories and increasing energy expenditure. Eating healthy foods and exercising are two proven ways to lose weight and keep it off.

Eat a Heart-Healthy Diet

When you have high blood pressure, heart health becomes very important. You will need to eat a balanced diet which focuses on fruit, vegetables, whole grains, and other kinds of food that are low in cholesterol, fat, and salt.

Supermarkets often have healthy sections where you can buy mayonnaise without fat, chips and nuts with less cholesterol, and sweet foods with no sugar added. These are good for your health and still taste delicious.

One of the more popular diets recommended by doctors to control high blood pressure is the DASH diet plan. We will discuss the DASH diet in the next chapter.

Exercise

Keep that body moving! Regular physical exercise lowers high blood pressure, keeps your heart strong, and helps you lose weight. The type and intensity of exercise you can do depends on the condition of your health. Before you embark on a workout plan, consult your doctor first.

Getting aerobic exercise and elevating heart levels at least three times per week for 20 minutes at a time is a great way to improve your heart health and physical condition. Whether you walk, hike, bike, run, jog, or take aerobic classes, you will enjoy the benefits of better health. You can also include strength training in your daily routine, but take care not to strain yourself in the process.

To keep exercise interesting, there are other workouts you can do. Yoga is a terrific way to relieve stress and dancing is a fun way to torch calories.

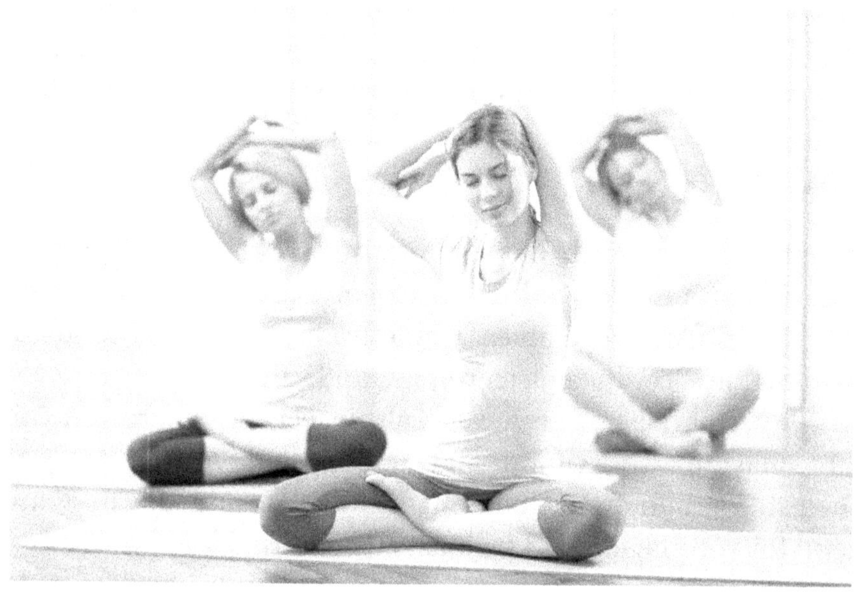

Reduce Sodium Intake

Many studies have shown that individuals who consume more salt have higher blood pressure. High sodium interferes with the body's fluid balance by holding excess water in the blood, causing elevated blood pressure, which puts extra strain on arteries and heart.

On average, Americans consume about 3,400 milligrams of salt per day, well above the American Heart Association's recommendation of 2,300 milligrams. Lowering one's sodium intake can significantly reduce high blood pressure. Here are a few suggestions for lowering salt consumption in your diet:

• A large portion of the sodium we eat comes from processed foods, so limit your intake of processed foods, including fast foods.

• Read the Daily Value (DV) of sodium on packaged foods. Foods with a sodium DV of 5% or less are considered low-sodium, while foods with more than 15% DV contain more sodium than your body needs.

• Avoid adding extra salt to your dishes. One teaspoon of salt contains about 2,300 mg sodium.

• Opt for foods with high potassium, such as vegetables and fruit, to counter the effects of sodium.

• Don't drastically cut your sodium intake, as it can have an adverse effect on your appetite. Reduce your sodium intake gradually.

Reduce Your Stress Levels

This one is, of course, a no-brainer. We all know how chronic stress contributes to an unhealthy body and mind. Bouts of stressful activities or anxiety can raise your blood pressure, causing you to feel restless. Take some time out to relax and prioritize your life. There's a chance you might have more on your plate than you can chew. Take occasional breaks from work and indulge in favorite activities like swimming and running, or treat yourself to some good food. Here are some more tips to help you reduce stress:

• Don't expect too much from yourself. Give yourself enough time to manage everything. Try not to control things when they change and accept it graciously.

• Make sure you are getting enough sleep each night. One of the biggest mistakes people make is to cut back on sleep with the hope of getting more done, but this often does not work and only leads to even more stress. Your body has to have a certain amount of sleep every night. Do not deprive yourself of sleep in some confused hope that it will help reduce stress.

• Identify your stress triggers. These may include heavy traffic, people who talk negatively, or constant criticism. Give yourself some time to figure out how you can start detaching from them.

• Take at least 15 minutes each day to practice deep breathing. You can also try some meditation techniques to quiet your mind.

• Expressing gratitude toward others can have a calming effect on you, thus helping you relieve your anxiety problems.

Get Support from Your Loved Ones

You may not realize this, but just being around loved ones can make a large difference in your overall health, and this includes blood pressure levels. When you are in the comforting company of those to whom you are close, your stress levels go down, and as a result, you are less likely to suffer from blood pressure fluctuations. You can also look for a social media support group that can provide you with a morale boost and offer you some valuable tips to improve your condition.

Quit Smoking

We all know how smoking is injurious to our health, but it is particularly harmful for your blood pressure levels. The nicotine in cigarettes raises blood pressure and heart rates. Long-term smoking may damage the arteries and harden artery walls. This is especially harmful to the cardiovascular system if you already have high blood pressure.

Quitting smoking is no easy feat. The following tips will help you stop it for good:

- Jot down the reasons why you want to quit. "It is bad for you" is often not enough motivation for people to quit. To be highly motivated, you need a powerful reminder to counteract the strong urge to smoke. Maybe the thought of stroke or lung cancer alarms you, or you want to limit your family's exposure to secondhand smoke. Whatever the reason, make sure it is something about which you are passionate.

- Don't quit cold turkey. You might be tempted to toss all of your cigarettes away and declare your resolve to quit smoking once and for all, but going cold turkey isn't as easy as it sounds. Over 95% of the people who try to suddenly stop smoking without any form of therapy or medication wind up relapsing, sooner rather than later. Without cigarettes, the body experiences nicotine withdrawal symptoms, such as headaches, drowsiness, anxiety, and irritability. Nicotine gum, patches, lozenges, or nicotine-rich prescription medications can help minimize nicotine withdrawal symptoms.

- Don't go it alone. Tell your family, friends, and even your co-workers about your plan to quit smoking. Their encouragement will help you succeed.

- Manage stress. One of the common reasons people smoke is to relieve stress. If you are planning on quitting, you need new ways to deal with stress. Yoga, listening to music, or massage sessions can help you deal with stress.

- Avoid all triggers. Some activities, including drinking alcohol, can trigger the urge to smoke, so try to limit alcohol when quitting smoking. If you are used to smoking after meals, find something else to do after meals, like take a walk or brush your teeth until the urge subsides.

- Don't give up. Most smokers relapse a few times before quitting for good. If you have a relapse, analyze the circumstances leading to the relapse, and use it as an opportunity to reaffirm your dedication to quit smoking for good, set a date, and try again.

Adopting lifestyle changes is not as easy as it sounds, but it's worth your best effort. A good strategy is to make one small, sustainable change at a time, and strive to get a little bit healthier every day. High blood pressure shouldn't stop you from living your life to the fullest!

Chapter 5: Introduction to the DASH Diet

The DASH diet was developed in line with medical research. The original intent of this eating program was to lower blood pressure. In fact, that's what DASH stands for: **D**ietary **A**pproaches to **S**top **H**ypertension. In addition to the benefit of lowering blood pressure, many people who follow the DASH diet lose weight because of the healthy foods the diet recommends.

A Brief History of the DASH Diet

In the mid-90s, large-scale studies were conducted at prestigious universities and medical centers to find new diet plans to help hypertension patients lower blood pressure. These studies, combined with follow-up studies and research, led to the development of the DASH diet plan. Today, the DASH diet is recommended by several important organizations, including the American Heart Association and the National Heart, Lung, and Blood Institute. The recommendations in this diet are the basis for U.S. Dietary Guidelines, and most doctors prescribe the DASH plan to patients who are battling high blood pressure. The DASH diet takes a scientific approach to good health, not by counting calories or measuring grams of fat, but with a holistic approach toward choosing the foods that are most likely to keep a body healthy.

Key Principles of the DASH Diet

The DASH diet focuses on long-term healthy eating habits. The diet doesn't force you to starve or battle constant cravings.

Instead, it focuses on understanding food groups, controlling portion sizes, and making sure you get the optimal levels of potassium, calcium, magnesium, fiber, and protein.

The diet focuses on certain food groups for specific reasons. Fruit and vegetables give you the magnesium and potassium your body needs, and low-fat dairy products provide calcium. Every food you eat should have a purpose, and that's the most important principle of the DASH diet: eat well so you feel well. Here are some additional points to remember when you're following the DASH principles:

Reduced Sodium Intake

The DASH diet as a whole aims to reduce sodium consumption. We've discussed that when you have too much sodium in your diet, it increases the risk for high blood pressure. The standard DASH diet recommends 2,300 milligrams of sodium a day. You can follow another version—called the low sodium Dash diet—which aims for 1,500 milligrams of sodium daily. The lower version is recommended for African Americans, for adults over 51, or for those with high blood pressure or diabetes.

Low Calorie

Vegetables and fruit are low in calories. The DASH diet's reduced servings of grains and fats also helps limit calorie consumption.

Low in Cholesterol

Since the DASH diet recommends small portions of lean meat, it is basically a low-fat diet. It is recommended you trim the skin and fat from chicken before cooking, and steam, bake, or broil instead of deep frying.

Low in Saturated Fats and Trans Fats

Saturated fats and trans fats are bad for our health in general. The DASH diet limits saturated and trans fats, and encourages healthy unsaturated fats.

Nutrient Rich and High in Fiber

Fiber binds cholesterol and prevents it from entering the bloodstream. The DASH diet plan provides all of the vitamins, minerals, and fiber we need to be healthy and manage blood pressure. Vegetables and fruit are high in fiber, potassium, magnesium, and vitamins A, B, C, D, and E. Dairy is rich in calcium and protein, while meat is a source of iron, protein, and zinc.

The DASH Diet for Lowering Blood Pressure

A major culprit of elevated blood pressure is salt—or sodium—and that's the target of the DASH diet: to eliminate excess sodium in your body and replace it with nutrients that are far more beneficial. Foods rich in potassium and magnesium have been found to help your body naturally reduce blood pressure. According to scientific studies, the DASH eating plan is just as effective as many blood pressure medications.

What to Eat on the DASH Diet

Healthy, high-fiber grains that are low in sugar are a great way to start on the DASH diet. These include whole grain cereals and breads, brown rice, and whole wheat pasta. Next, aim for four or five servings of fruit and vegetables every day. Recommended vegetables include lettuce, cabbage, celery, carrots, spinach, squash, broccoli, cucumbers, tomatoes, and mushrooms. Recommended fruit includes blackberries, blueberries, strawberries, apples, pears, bananas, avocados, citrus fruit, melons, and mangos.

You can have milk, yogurt, and cheese, too, just be sure to watch out for added salt and sugar in these products. Nuts and legumes are also a big part of the DASH diet. Get your protein from beans, eggs, and lean meats. In addition, the DASH diet encourages fish, such as salmon, tilapia, and mackerel.

Transitioning to the DASH Diet

Changing your eating habits needs to be done gradually. Here are a few suggestions to help you make an easy transition to the DASH diet:

• Keep a journal and track your eating habits. What do you eat for breakfast, lunch, and dinner? How often do you eat in between meals, and on what are you snacking? Figure out where you need to make changes from your journal. For example, add a cup or two of vegetables and fruit to help reduce too many servings of meat. Limit your sodium and sugar by reading the nutrition fact labels on food packages.

• When shopping, choose low-fat, non-fat, no sugar added, no cholesterol, and other, healthier versions of products. For grain servings, choose whole grains, such as whole wheat bread and whole grain cereals.

• If you love butter or margarine, decrease the amount you use by half and switch to no cholesterol and low-sodium versions. You can use spices as a substitute for salt. Experiment with different herbs if you're not sure how they taste. Some examples of spices you can try are rosemary, basil, nutmeg, parsley, sage, and thyme.

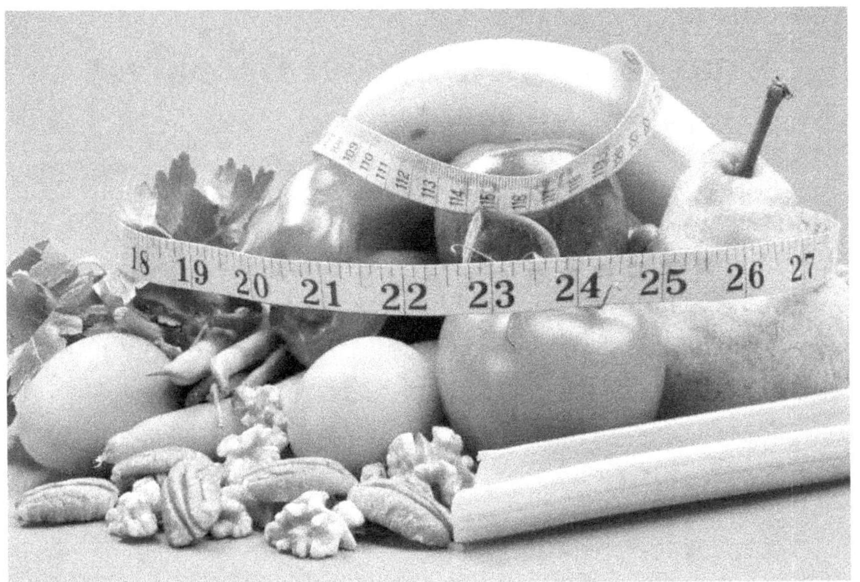

The 32 delicious DASH diet recipes in the following chapters will help you make dietary changes, lower your blood pressure, and lose weight.

Chapter 6: DASH Diet Breakfast Recipes

These breakfast recipes follow the DASH diet plan for lowering your blood pressure. The meals are full of fruits, vegetables, whole grains, and healthy dairy products. Start the day off with one of these scrumptious meals and you'll reduce your risk for cardiovascular problems and weight gain.

Oat Smoothie

Yield: 4 servings
Preparation Time: 10 minutes
Total Time: 35 minutes
Ingredients:
2/3 cups rolled oats
2 oranges, peeled, seeded, and sectioned
2 large bananas, peeled and sliced
2 cups unsweetened almond milk
1 cup ice cubes, crushed

Directions:
1. In a high speed blender, add rolled oats and pulse until finely chopped.
2. Add remaining ingredients and pulse until smooth.
3. Transfer into 4 serving glasses and serve immediately.

Nutritional Information (Per Serving)
Calories: 175
Fat: 3g
Sat Fat: 0.4g
Carbohydrates: 36.6g
Fiber: 5.9g

Sugar: 17.1g
Protein: 3.9g
Sodium: 93mg

Berry Bowl

Yield: 2 servings
Preparation Time: 15 minutes
Total Time: 15 minutes
Ingredients:
2 cups frozen blueberries
1/3 cup unsweetened almond milk
¼ cup fat-free plain Greek yogurt
2 tablespoons unsweetened whey protein powder
¼ cup fresh blueberries

Directions:
1. In a blender, add blueberries and pulse for about 1 minute.
2. Add almond milk, yogurt, and protein powder and pulse until desired consistency.
3. Transfer the mixture into 2 serving bowls, dividing evenly.
4. Serve topped with fresh blueberries.

Nutritional Information (Per Serving)
Calories: 160
Fat: 1.8g
Sat Fat: 0.2g
Carbohydrates: 23.5g
Fiber: 3.7g
Sugar: 16.1g
Protein: 15.3g
Sodium: 70mg

French Toasts Casserole

Yield: 2 servings
Preparation Time: 10 minutes
Cooking Time: 2 minutes
Total Time: 12 minutes
Ingredients:

2 whole-wheat bread slices, cubed

2 teaspoons unsalted margarine, softened

1 cup egg whites, slightly beaten

2 tablespoons applesauce

2 tablespoons almonds, chopped

Directions:

1. In a microwave safe bowl, mix the cubed bread and margarine.

2. Top with egg whites evenly and drizzle with applesauce.

3. Microwave on high for about 1 minute.

4. Remove from microwave and push away the edges of egg whites with a spoon.

5. Microwave for about 1 minute more.

6. Remove from microwave and divide into 2 portions.

7. Serve warm, topped with almonds.

Nutritional Information (Per Serving)

Calories: 207

Fat: 7.9g

Sat Fat: 1.1g

Carbohydrates: 15.5g

Fiber: 2.8g

Sugar: 4.2g

Protein: 18.2g

Sodium: 299mg

Veggie Scramble

Yield: 4 servings
Preparation Time: 15 minutes
Cooking Time: 20 minutes
Total Time: 35 minutes
Ingredients:
½ cup chickpea flour
2 tablespoons nutritional yeast
2 teaspoons mustard
¼ teaspoon paprika
¼ teaspoon ground turmeric
1/8 teaspoon ground cumin
Freshly ground black pepper to taste
1/3 cup water
1½ cups cooked chickpeas
2 tablespoons fresh parsley, chopped
1 garlic clove, minced
1 tablespoon olive oil
½ bell pepper, seeded and chopped
½ onion, chopped
1 cup cherry tomatoes, halved

Directions:
1. In food processor, add chickpea flour, nutritional yeast, mustard, spices, and black pepper and pulse until well combined.

2. With motor slowly running, add water and mix until smooth mixture forms.

3. Add chickpeas and pulse until finely chopped.

4. Add parsley and garlic and mix well.

5. In a large skillet, heat oil on medium-high heat.

6. Add bell pepper and onion and sauté for about 5-6 minutes.

7. Add chickpea mixture and cook, stirring continuously for about 3-4 minutes.

8. Add tomatoes and reduce heat to medium.

9. Cook for about 10 minutes, turning tomatoes at the five-minute mark.

Nutritional Information (Per Serving)
Calories: 235
Fat: 7g
Sat Fat: 0.6g
Carbohydrates: 34g
Fiber: 10.2g
Sugar: 7.3g
Protein: 12g
Sodium: 17mg

Oat & Nut Granola

Yield: 22 servings
Preparation Time: 15 minutes
Cooking Time: 25 minutes
Total Time: 40 minutes
Ingredients:
¼ cup applesauce
¼ cup canola oil
1½ teaspoons vanilla extract
6 cups old-fashioned rolled oats
2 cups bran flakes
1 cup almonds, slivered
¾ cup walnuts, chopped
½ cup unsweetened coconut, shredded
1 cup raisins

Directions:
1. Preheat oven to 325 degrees F. Lightly grease a baking sheet.
2. In a small pan over low heat, add applesauce, oil, and vanilla extract.
3. Cook for about 5 minutes, stirring occasionally.
4. Add remaining ingredients except for raisins and stir gently to combine.
5. Transfer the mixture onto prepared baking sheet.
6. Bake for about 25 minutes or until golden brown, stirring occasionally.
7. Remove from oven and set aside to cool.
8. Add raisins and stir to combine.
9. Granola may be preserved in airtight container.

Nutritional Information (Per Serving)
Calories: 197
Fat: 9.5g

Sat Fat: 1.3g
Carbohydrates: 25g
Fiber: 4.1g
Sugar: 5.9g
Protein: 5.3g
Sodium: 28mg

Quinoa Porridge

Yield: 4 servings
Preparation Time: 15 minutes
Cooking Time: 25 minutes
Total Time: 40 minutes
Ingredients:
2 cups unsweetened soy milk
1 cup uncooked quinoa, rinsed
¼ teaspoon vanilla extract
Pinch of ground cinnamon
1 date, pitted and chopped very finely
1 cup banana, peeled and sliced

Directions:
1. In a pan, combine milk, quinoa, vanilla, and cinnamon on low heat.
2. Cook, stirring occasionally for about 15-20 minutes.
3. Remove from heat and stir in chopped date.
4. Top with banana slices and serve.

Nutritional Information (Per Serving)
Calories: 263
Fat: 4.9g
Sat Fat: 0.6g
Carbohydrates: 45.2g
Fiber: 4.9g
Sugar: 10.8g
Protein: 10.5g
Sodium: 65mg

Mushroom Muffins

Yield: 6 servings
Preparation Time: 15 minutes
Cooking Time: 30 minutes
Total Time: 45 minutes
Ingredients:
1 teaspoon olive oil
1½ cups fresh mushrooms, chopped
1 scallion, chopped
1 teaspoon garlic, minced
1 teaspoon fresh rosemary, minced
Freshly ground black pepper to taste
1 (12.3-ounce) package lite, firm, silken tofu, drained
¼ cup unsweetened soy milk
2 tablespoons nutritional yeast
1 tablespoon arrowroot starch
1 teaspoon unsalted butter, softened
¼ teaspoon ground turmeric

Directions:
1. Preheat oven to 375 degrees F. Grease a 12-cup muffin pan.
2. In a nonstick skillet, heat oil on medium heat.
3. Add scallion and garlic and sauté for about 1 minute.
4. Add mushrooms and sauté for about 5-7 minutes.
5. Stir in rosemary and black pepper and remove from the heat.
6. Keep aside to cool slightly.
7. In a food processor, add tofu and remaining ingredients and pulse until smooth.
8. Transfer tofu mixture into a large bowl.
9. Fold in mushroom mixture.
10. Spoon mixture evenly into prepared muffin cups.

11. Bake for about 20-22 minutes or until a toothpick inserted in center comes out clean.

12. Remove muffin pan from oven and place on wire rack to cool for about 10 minutes.

13. Carefully, invert muffins onto wire rack and serve warm.

Nutritional Information (Per Serving)
Calories: 88
Fat: 4.2g
Sat Fat: 1g
Carbohydrates: 7.3g
Fiber: 1.4g
Sugar: 1.9g
Protein: 7.2g
Sodium: 21mg

Chicken Quiche

Yield: 8 servings
Preparation Time: 15 minutes
Cooking Time: 45 minutes
Total Time: 1 hour
Ingredients:
1 teaspoon olive oil
½ cup onion, sliced
2 garlic cloves, minced
3 cups small broccoli florets
2 cups cooked chicken, chopped
2 large eggs
4 large egg whites
1¼ cups fat-free milk
1 cup fat-free Cheddar cheese, shredded
Freshly ground black pepper to taste
1 tablespoon low-fat Parmesan cheese, shredded

Directions:
1. Preheat oven to 350 degrees F. Grease a 9-inch pie plate.
2. In a skillet, heat oil on medium heat.
3. Add onion and garlic and sauté for about 2-3 minutes.
4. Add broccoli and chicken and sauté for about 1-2 minutes.
5. Transfer mixture to prepared pie dish.
6. In a bowl, add eggs, egg whites, milk, cheddar cheese, salt, and black pepper and beat until well-combined.
7. Pour egg mixture over chicken mixture and top with Parmesan cheese.
8. Bake for about 40 minutes or until top is golden brown.
9. Remove from oven. Cut into 8 equal-sized wedges and serve.

Nutritional Information (Per Serving)

Calories: 190
Fat: 7.9g
Sat Fat: 3.8g
Carbohydrates: 7.7g
Fiber: 1g
Sugar: 5.3g
Protein: 2.1g
Sodium: 210mg

Chapter 7: DASH Diet Lunch Recipes

When you're looking for DASH diet lunch recipes, you're looking for food that's healthy but filling. There are many fruits, vegetables, whole grains, and lean proteins that combine to make fresh, tasty, and healthful meals that you can eat at home or at work. These recipes will give you a bolt of energy in the middle of the day and feed your body with the vitamins, nutrients, and ingredients that it really needs and craves.

Cabbage and Broccoli Salad

Yield: 4 servings
Preparation Time: 15 minutes
Total Time: 15 minutes
Ingredients:
For Dressing:
1 tablespoon shallot, minced
1/3 cup of olive oil
2 tablespoons fresh lemon juice
3 drops liquid stevia
Freshly ground black pepper to taste

For Salad:
1¼ cup broccoli florets, chopped
1¼ cups cabbage, shredded
6 cups romaine lettuce, chopped

Directions:
1. In a bowl, add all dressing ingredients and beat until well combined. Keep aside.
2. In another large bowl, mix all salad ingredients together.

3. Add dressing and toss gently to coat well.
4. Serve immediately.

Nutritional Information (Per Serving)
Calories: 174
Fat: 17.1g
Sat Fat: 2.5g
Carbohydrates: 6.2g
Fiber: 1.9g
Sugar: 2.2g
Protein: 1.6g
Sodium: 20mg

Vegetable Sandwich

Yield: 4 servings
Preparation Time: 15 minutes
Total Time: 15 minutes
Ingredients:
1 avocado, peeled, pitted, and chopped
1 large tomato, sliced
½ cup red onion, sliced thinly
8 romaine lettuce leaves, chopped
8 whole wheat bread slices, toasted
¼ cup Dijon mustard

Directions:
1. In a large bowl, mix avocado, tomato, onion, and lettuce.
2. Evenly divide and spread Dijon mustard on each slice.
3. Evenly divide and place avocado mixture over 4 slices.
4. Cover with remaining slices.
5. With a knife, carefully cut sandwiches diagonally and serve.

Nutritional Information (Per Serving)
Calories: 267
Fat: 12.4g
Sat Fat: 2.5g
Carbohydrates: 31.7g
Fiber: 31.7g
Sugar: 5.4g
Protein: 9.5g
Sodium: 440mg

Turkey Lettuce Wraps

Yield: 4 servings
Preparation Time: 25 minutes
Cooking Time: 20 minutes
Total Time: 45 minutes
Ingredients:
1 tablespoon olive oil
1 cup onion, chopped
¾ pound lean ground turkey
1 cup fresh mushrooms, chopped
½ tablespoon fresh ginger, minced
1 tablespoon soy sauce
½ tablespoon cayenne pepper
½ tablespoon ground cumin
8 large romaine lettuce leaves
2 tablespoons fresh cilantro leaves, chopped

Directions:
1. In a skillet, heat oil on medium heat.
2. Add onion and sauté for about 4-5 minutes.
3. Add turkey and cook for about 6-8 minutes, stirring occasionally.
4. Add mushroom, ginger, tamari, cayenne pepper, and cumin and cook for about 5-7 minutes.
5. Remove from heat and set aside.
6. Arrange lettuce leaves onto serving plates.
7. Place turkey mixture over each lettuce leaf evenly.
8. Top with cilantro and serve.

Nutritional Information (Per Serving)
Calories: 174
Fat: 9.6g
Sat Fat: 2.4g
Carbohydrates: 4.8g

Fiber: 1.2g
Sugar: 0.4g
Protein: 18.1g
Sodium: 317mg

Bean Burgers

Yield: 6 servings
Preparation Time: 20 minutes
Cooking Time: 25 minutes
Total Time: 45 minutes
Ingredients:
½ cup walnuts
1 carrot, peeled and chopped
1 celery stalk, chopped
4 scallions, chopped
5 garlic cloves, chopped
2¼ cups cooked black beans
2½ cups sweet potato, peeled and grated
½ teaspoon red pepper flakes, crushed
Freshly ground black pepper to taste
10 cups fresh baby spinach
½ cup fresh pomegranate seeds

Directions:
1. Preheat the oven to 400 degrees F. Line a baking sheet with parchment paper.

2. Add walnuts to food processor, until finely ground.

3. Add carrot, celery, scallion, and garlic and pulse until finely chopped.

4. Transfer vegetable mixture to large bowl.

5. In same food processor, add beans and pulse until chopped.

6. Add 1½ cups sweet potato and pulse until chunky mixture forms.

7. Transfer bean mixture into bowl with vegetable mixture.

8. Stir in remaining sweet potato and spices and mix until well combined.

9. Make 8 patties from mixture.

10. Arrange patties on prepared baking sheet in a single layer.

11. Bake for about 25 minutes.

12. Divide spinach and pomegranate seeds evenly into 8 servings. Place each serving on a plate.

13. Top each plate with 1 burger and serve.

Nutritional Information (Per Serving)
Calories: 326
Fat: 5.9g
Sat Fat: 0.5g
Carbohydrates: 55.1g
Fiber: 13g
Sugar: 9.1g
Protein: 16.6g
Sodium: 64mg

Chicken Kabobs

Yield: 10 servings
Preparation Time: 20 minutes
Cooking Time: 12 minutes
Total Time: 32 minutes
Ingredients:

3 tablespoons low-sodium soy sauce

2 tablespoons applesauce

3 tablespoons balsamic vinegar

2 tablespoons olive oil

3 tablespoons fresh ginger, chopped

3 tablespoons fresh garlic, chopped

1 teaspoon red pepper flakes, crushed

3 cups skinless, boneless chicken, cubed

2½ cups fresh pineapple cubes

2 red bell peppers, seeded and cubed

Directions:

1. In a large bowl, mix soy sauce, applesauce, vinegar, oil, ginger, garlic, and red pepper flakes.

2. Add the chicken and generously coat with marinade.

3. Cover and refrigerate for about 2-3 hours.

4. Preheat grill to medium-high heat. Grease grill grate.

5. Thread chicken, pineapple, and bell pepper onto skewers.

6. Grill for about 10-12 minutes or until desired doneness, flipping occasionally.

Nutritional Information (Per Serving)

Calories: 129

Fat: 4.3g

Sat Fat: 0.8g

Carbohydrates: 10g

Fiber: 1.2g

Sugar: 6g
Protein: 13.3g
Sodium: 293mg

Stuffed Bell Peppers

Yield: 4 servings
Preparation Time: 15 minutes
Cooking Time: 25 minutes
Total Time: 40 minutes
Ingredients:
½ pound shiitake mushrooms
1 cup celery stalk
2 garlic cloves, peeled
½ cup walnuts, chopped
2 tablespoons olive oil
Pinch of salt
Freshly ground black pepper to taste
4 small red bell peppers, halved and seeded

Directions:
1. Preheat oven to 400 degrees F. Grease baking sheet.
2. Remove stem and seeds from bell peppers.
3. In food processor, add mushrooms, celery, garlic, walnuts, oil, salt, and pepper and pulse until finely chopped.
4. Stuff bell peppers with mushroom mixture.
5. Arrange bell peppers onto prepared baking sheet.
6. Bake for about 20-25 minutes.

Nutritional Information (Per Serving)
Calories: 232
Fat: 16.7g
Sat Fat: 1.6g
Carbohydrates: 19.6g
Fiber: 4.3g
Sugar: 8.6g
Protein: 6.1g
Sodium: 199mg

Broccoli with Apple

Yield: 4 servings
Preparation Time: 15 minutes
Cooking Time: 17 minutes
Total Time: 32 minutes
Ingredients:
1 tablespoon olive oil
2 garlic cloves, minced
2 cups small broccoli florets
½ cup red onion, chopped
¼ cup celery stalk, chopped
¼ cup low-sodium vegetable broth
2 apples, cored and sliced

Directions:
1. In a large skillet, heat oil on medium-high heat.
2. Add garlic and sauté for about 1 minute.
3. Add broccoli and stir fry for about 4-5 minutes.
4. Add celery and onion and stir fry for about 4-5 minutes.
5. Stir in broth and cook for about 2-3 minutes.
6. Add apple slices and cook for about 2-3 minutes.
7. Serve hot.

Nutritional Information (Per Serving)
Calories: 105
Fat: 3.7g
Sat Fat: 0.5g
Carbohydrates: 18.6g
Fiber: 3.9g
Sugar: 12.7g
Protein: 1.1g
Sodium: 56mg

Green Beans and Tomato Combo

Yield: 6 servings
Preparation Time: 15 minutes
Cooking Time: 17 minutes
Total Time: 32 minutes
Ingredients:
2 teaspoons olive oil
¼ teaspoon fresh lemon peel, finely grated
Pinch of freshly ground white pepper
3 cups grape tomatoes
2 pounds fresh green beans, trimmed
1 tablespoon fresh parsley, chopped

Directions:
1. Preheat the oven to 350 degrees F.
2. In large bowl, mix lemon peel, oil, and white pepper.
3. Add cherry tomatoes and toss until well-coated.
4. Transfer tomato mixture to a roasting pan.
5. Roast for about 35-40 minutes, stirring once in half-way through.
6. Meanwhile, place steamer basket in a pan of boiling water.
7. Place green beans in steamer basket. Cover and steam for about 7-8 minutes. Drain well.
8. Divide green beans and tomatoes and place on serving plates.
9. Sprinkle with parsley and serve hot.

Nutritional Information (Per Serving)
Calories: 77
Fat: 1.9g
Sat Fat: 0.3g
Carbohydrates: 14.4g
Fiber: 6.3g

Sugar: 4.5g
Protein: 3.6g
Sodium: 17mg

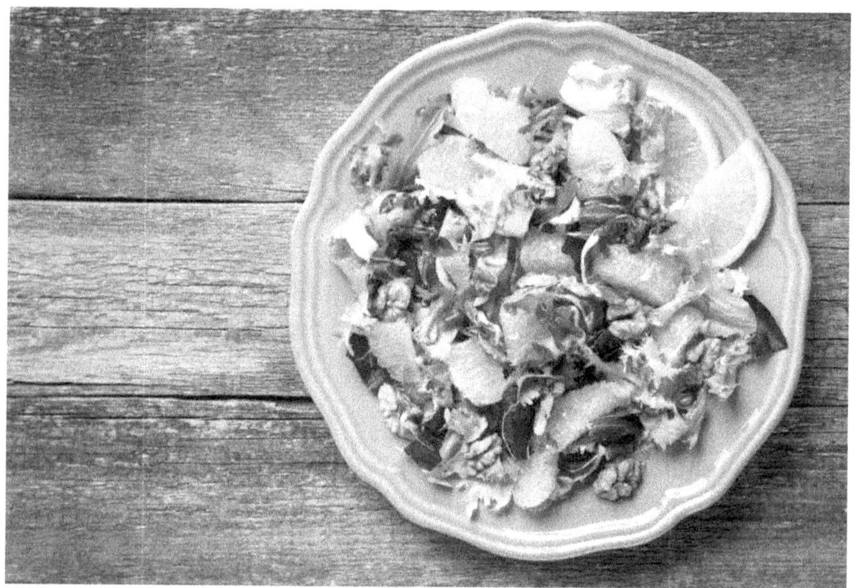

Chapter 8: DASH Diet Snack Recipes

Roasted Chickpeas

Yield: 4 servings
Preparation Time: 10 minutes
Cooking Time: 30 minutes
Total Time: 40 minutes
Ingredients:
1 (15-ounce) can low-sodium chickpeas, rinsed and drained
1 tablespoon extra-virgin olive oil
1 teaspoon dried marjoram, crushed
1 teaspoon ground cumin
½ teaspoon cayenne pepper
¼ teaspoon ground allspice

Directions:
1. Preheat oven to 450 degrees F. Arrange rack in upper third of the oven.
2. Pat chickpeas dry with paper towels. Add oil, marjoram, and spices and toss to coat.
3. Spread chickpeas onto rimmed baking sheet.
4. Bake for about 25-30 minutes, stirring once mid-way through.
5. Remove from oven and set aside to cool on baking sheet for about 15 minutes.

Nutritional Information (Per Serving)
Calories: 147
Fat: 6g
Sat Fat: 0.9g
Carbohydrates: 16.7g
Fiber: 5.2g

Sugar: 0.6g
Protein: 7.1g
Sodium: 0.2mg

Deviled Eggs

Yield: 6 servings
Preparation Time: 15 minutes
Cooking Time: 20 minutes
Total Time: 35 minutes
Ingredients:
6 large eggs
1 medium avocado, peeled, pitted, and chopped
2 teaspoons fresh lime juice
Pinch of salt
1/8 teaspoon cayenne pepper

Directions:
1. In a pot of water, hard boil eggs, cooking for about 15-20 minutes.
2. Drain water and let eggs cool completely.
3. Peel eggs and slice in half vertically with sharp knife.
4. Scoop out yolks and transfer half of them to bowl.
5. Add avocado, lime juice, and salt and mash with fork until well combined.
5. Fill egg halves with avocado mixture.
6. Sprinkle with cayenne pepper and serve.

Nutritional Information (Per Serving)
Calories: 140
Fat: 11.5g
Sat Fat: 2.9g
Carbohydrates: 3.3g
Fiber: 2.3g
Sugar: 0.6g
Protein: 6.9g
Sodium: 99mg

Tomato Bruschetta

Yield: 6 servings
Preparation Time: 15 minutes
Cooking Time: 4 minutes
Total Time: 19 minutes
Ingredients:
½ whole-grain baguette, cut into 6 (½-inch-thick) slices on the diagonal
3 tomatoes, chopped
½ cup fennel, chopped
2 garlic cloves, minced
1 tablespoon fresh parsley, chopped
1 tablespoon fresh basil, chopped
2 teaspoons balsamic vinegar
1 teaspoon olive oil
Freshly ground black pepper to taste

Directions:
1. Preheat the oven to broil. Arrange rack in top portion of oven.

2. Arrange bread slices on baking sheet in single layer.

3. Broil for about 2 minutes per side.

4. Meanwhile, in bowl, add remaining ingredients and toss to coat.

5. Divide tomato mixture evenly and place on each slice of toasted bread. Serve immediately.

Nutritional Information (Per Serving)
Calories: 94.5
Fat: 1.5g
Sat Fat: 0.1g
Carbohydrates: 18g
Fiber: 2.5g
Sugar: 1.0g

Protein: 3.7g
Sodium: 176mg

Apple Cookies

Yield: 7 servings
Preparation Time: 15 minutes
Cooking Time: 15 minutes
Total Time: 30 minutes
Ingredients:

1 cup instant oats

¾ cup whole wheat flour

1½ teaspoons baking powder

1 teaspoon ground cinnamon

¼ teaspoon ground ginger

Pinch of ground cloves

Pinch of salt

1 large egg

½ cup applesauce

2 tablespoons unsalted butter, melted

1 teaspoon vanilla extract

1 cup apple, peeled, cored, and finely chopped

Directions:

1. In a bowl, mix together oats, flour, baking powder, spices, and salt.

2. Add remaining ingredients to a second large bowl except for apple and beat until well combined.

3. Add flour mixture to egg mixture and mix until just combined.

4. Fold apple in gently.

5. Chill in refrigerator for about 30 minutes.

6. Preheat oven to 325 degrees F. Line a cookie sheet with parchment paper.

7. With tablespoon, place mixture onto prepared cookie sheet in a single layer.

8. Flatten each cookie slightly using hands.

9. Bake for about 13-15 minutes.

10. Remove from oven and keep on wire rack to cool in pan for about 10 minutes.

11. Carefully turn onto wire rack until completely cooled.

Nutritional Information (Per Serving)
Calories: 140
Fat: 4.7g
Sat Fat: 2.4g
Carbohydrates: 21.6g
Fiber: 2.1g
Sugar: 5.4g
Protein: 3.3g
Sodium: 60mg

Chapter 9: DASH Diet Dinner Recipes

When the dinner bell rings, it's time to fill up on delicious comfort food that won't compromise your health goals. Whether you're setting a table for one or calling the entire family to the table, make sure you have something good to serve. These DASH diet dinner recipes aren't complicated or time consuming. Make a little extra if you want to have leftovers for lunch the next day.

Chickpeas and Barley Soup

Yield: 8 servings
Preparation Time: 20 minutes
Cooking Time: 1½ hours
Total Time: 1 hour 50 minutes
Ingredients:
1 cup dry barley
1 (15-ounce) can low-sodium chickpeas, rinsed and drained
2 large carrots, peeled and chopped
1 zucchini, chopped
2 celery stalks, chopped
1 onion, chopped
2 cups tomatoes, chopped
1 teaspoon dried parsley, crushed
1 teaspoon curry powder
1 teaspoon paprika
3 bay leaves
Freshly ground black pepper to taste
5 cups low-sodium vegetable broth
4 cups water
½ cup fresh cilantro, chopped

Directions:

1. In large soup pan, add all ingredients except for parsley and bring to a boil on high heat.

2. Reduce heat to medium-low. Cover and simmer for about 1½ hours.

3. Discard bay leaf before serving.

4. Serve hot, garnishing with cilantro.

Nutritional Information (Per Serving)

Calories: 312

Fat: 4g

Sat Fat: 0.5g

Carbohydrates: 55.9g

Fiber: 15.1g

Sugar: 9.1g

Protein: 15.5g

Sodium: 85mg

Vegetable Stew

Yield: 5 servings
Preparation Time: 20 minutes
Cooking Time: 25 minutes
Total Time: 45 minutes
Ingredients:
2 tablespoons olive oil
1 large onion, chopped
2 garlic cloves, minced
¼ teaspoon fresh ginger, finely grated
1 teaspoon ground cumin
1 teaspoon cayenne pepper
Freshly ground black pepper to taste
2 cups low-sodium vegetable broth
1½ cups small broccoli florets
1 cup cabbage, shredded
2 large carrots, peeled and sliced
1 teaspoon fresh lemon zest, finely grated

Directions:
1. In a large soup pan, heat oil on medium heat.
2. Add onion and sauté for about 3-4 minutes.
3. Add garlic, turmeric, ginger, and spices and sauté for about 1 minute.
4. Add 1 cup of broth and bring to a boil.
5. Add vegetables and bring to boil once more.
6. Cover and simmer for about 15-20 minutes, stirring occasionally.
7. Serve hot, topped with lemon zest.

Nutritional Information (Per Serving)
Calories: 96
Fat: 5.9g
Sat Fat: 0.8g

Carbohydrates: 9.6g
Fiber: 2.6g
Sugar: 3.7g
Protein: 2.5g
Sodium: 62mg

Salmon Curry

Yield: 4 servings
Preparation Time: 15 minutes
Cooking Time: 15 minutes
Total Time: 30 minutes
Ingredients:
1 tablespoon olive oil
1 small onion, chopped
2 garlic cloves, minced
1 teaspoon fresh ginger, minced
1 large tomatoes, peeled and chopped
½ tablespoon curry powder
¼ cup water
1¼ cups fat-free plain Greek yogurt, whipped
1½ pounds skinless salmon fillets cut into 2-inch cubes
¼ cup fresh parsley, chopped

Directions:
1. In a large skillet, heat oil on medium heat.
2. Add onion, garlic, and ginger and sauté for about 3-4 minutes.
3. Add tomatoes and cook for about 2-3 minutes, crushing with back of spoon.
4. Add curry paste and sauté for about 2 minutes.
5. Add water and yogurt and bring to a gentle boil.
6. Stir in salmon and cook for about 5-6 minutes or until desired doneness.
7. Serve hot, garnished with parsley.

Nutritional Information (Per Serving)
Calories: 322
Fat: 14.5g
Sat Fat: 2g
Carbohydrates: 8g

Fiber: 1.4g
Sugar: 4.8g
Protein: 41.4g
Sodium: 117mg

Lentil and Spinach Chili

Yield: 8 servings
Preparation Time: 15 minutes
Cooking Time: 2 hours 10 minutes
Total Time: 2 hours 25 minutes
Ingredients:
2 teaspoons olive oil
1 large onion, chopped
3 medium carrot, peeled and chopped
4 celery stalks, chopped
2 garlic cloves, minced
1 jalapeño pepper, seeded and chopped
½ tablespoon dried thyme, crushed
1 tablespoon chipotle chili powder
½ tablespoon cayenne pepper
1½ tablespoons ground coriander
1½ tablespoons ground cumin
1 teaspoon ground turmeric
Freshly ground black pepper to taste
2 tablespoons tomato paste
1 pound lentils, rinsed
8 cups low-sodium vegetable broth
6 cups fresh spinach
½ cup fresh cilantro, chopped
½ cup sour cream

Directions:
1. In a large pan, heat oil on medium.
2. Add onion, carrot, and celery and sauté for about 5 minutes.
3. Add garlic, jalapeño pepper, thyme, and spices and sauté for about 1 minute.
4. Add tomato paste, lentils, and broth and bring to a boil.
5. Reduce heat to low and simmer for about 2 hours.

6. Stir in spinach and simmer for about 3-4 minutes.
7. Stir in cilantro and remove from heat.
8. Serve hot, topped with sour cream.

Nutritional Information (Per Serving)
Calories: 309
Fat: 6.1g
Sat Fat: 2.3g
Carbohydrates: 44.8g
Fiber: 20.1g
Sugar: 4.1g
Protein: 19.4g
Sodium: 144mg

Stuffed Chicken Breast

Yield: 4 servings
Preparation Time: 15 minutes
Cooking Time: 24 minutes
Total Time: 39 minutes
Ingredients:

4 (4-ounce) skinless, boneless chicken breast halves, pounded to ½-inch thickness
Pinch of salt
Freshly ground black pepper to taste
¼ cup Kalamata olives, pitted and chopped
¼ cup oil packed sun-dried tomatoes, drained
¼ cup feta cheese, crumbled
1 tablespoon fresh dill, chopped
1 tablespoon fresh parsley, chopped
1 tablespoon olive oil

Directions:

1. Preheat oven to 375 degrees F. Grease a rimmed baking sheet.

2. Rub chicken with pinch of salt and black pepper.

3. In a large bowl, mix olives, tomatoes, feta cheese, scallion, dill, and parsley.

4. Place chicken breast on cutting board.

5. Stuff chicken breasts with olive mixture and roll tightly.

6. Secure each roll with toothpicks.

7. In a skillet, heat oil on medium-high heat.

8. Add chicken breast rolls and cook for about 2 minutes per side.

9. Arrange the chicken breast on prepared baking sheet in a single layer.

10. Bake for about 15-20 minutes or until desired doneness.

11. Remove from oven and set aside for about 5 minutes.

12. With a sharp knife, cut into slices and serve.

Nutritional Information (Per Serving)
Calories: 223
Fat: 11.5g
Sat Fat: 3.7g
Carbohydrates: 3g
Fiber: 0.8g
Sugar: 0.4g
Protein: 27.3g
Sodium: 278mg

Turkey with Peas

Yield: 5 servings
Preparation Time: 15 minutes
Cooking Time: 40 minutes
Total Time: 55 minutes
Ingredients:
1 tablespoon olive oil
1 medium onion, chopped
½ teaspoon fresh ginger, minced
4 garlic cloves, minced
1½ teaspoons ground coriander
½ teaspoon ground cumin
½ teaspoon ground turmeric
¼ teaspoon ground nutmeg
2 bay leaves
1 pound lean ground turkey
½ cup fresh tomatoes, chopped
1-1½ cups water
1 cup fresh green peas, shelled
Pinch of salt
Freshly ground black pepper to taste
¼ cup fresh cilantro, chopped

Directions:
1. In a large pan, heat oil on medium-high heat.
2. Add onion and sauté for about 3-4 minutes.
3. Add ginger, garlic cloves, and spices and sauté for about 1 minute.
4. Add turkey and cook for about 5 minutes.
5. Add tomatoes and cook for about 10 minutes.
6. Stir in water and green peas. Cover and cook for about 25-30 minutes.
7. Stir in salt and black pepper. Remove from heat when desired doneness.

8. Serve hot, garnishing with cilantro.

Nutritional Information (Per Serving)
Calories: 196
Fat: 9.6g
Sat Fat: 2.5g
Carbohydrates: 8.2g
Fiber: 2.4g
Sugar: 3.1g
Protein: 20g
Sodium: 107mg

Tilapia with Veggies

Yield: 2 servings
Preparation Time: 20 minutes
Cooking Time: 25 minutes
Total Time: 45 minutes
Ingredients:
2 (3-ounce) tilapia fillets
1 cup zucchini, sliced
1 cup summer squash, sliced
1 cup tomato, sliced
1 cup red bell pepper, seeded and sliced
1 cup red onion, sliced
2 tablespoons fresh rosemary, minced
Pinch of salt
Freshly ground black pepper to taste
3 teaspoons olive oil

Directions:
1. Preheat the oven to 350 degrees F. Grease a large baking dish.
2. Place all ingredients except for oil in large bowl and toss to coat.
3. Transfer mixture into prepared baking dish.
4. Bake for about 20-25 minutes.
5. Transfer mixture to serving plate.
6. Drizzle with oil and serve.

Nutritional Information (Per Serving)
Calories: 220
Fat: 8.9g
Sat Fat: 1.7g
Carbohydrates: 19.9g
Fiber: 5.8g
Sugar: 11g

Protein: 19.3g
Sodium: 152mg

Rice and Lentil Casserole

Yield: 6 servings
Preparation Time: 20 minutes
Cooking Time: 1 hour 20 minutes
Total Time: 1 hour 40 minutes
Ingredients:
2½ cups water, divided
1 cup red lentils
½ cup wild rice
1 teaspoon olive oil
1 small onion, chopped
3 garlic cloves, minced
1/3 cup zucchini, chopped
1/3 cup carrot, peeled and chopped
1/3 cup celery stalk, chopped
1 fresh tomato, chopped
8-ounce low-sodium tomato sauce
1 teaspoon ground cumin
1 teaspoon dried oregano, crushed
1 teaspoon dried basil, crushed
Freshly ground black pepper to taste

Directions:
1. In a pan, add rice and 1 cup of water and bring to boil on medium heat.

2. Reduce heat to low, cover, and simmer for about 20 minutes.

3. Meanwhile, in another pan, add remaining water and lentils and bring to boil on medium heat.

4. Reduce heat to low, cover, and simmer, for about 15 minutes.

5. Transfer cooked rice and lentils to casserole dish and set aside.

6. Preheat oven to 350 degrees F.

7. In large skillet, heat oil on medium heat.

8. Add onion and garlic and sauté for about 4-5 minutes.

9. Add zucchini, carrots, celery, tomato, and tomato paste and cook for about 4-5 minutes.

10. Stir in cumin, herbs, salt, and black pepper and remove from heat.

11. Transfer vegetable mixture into casserole dish with rice and lentils and stir to combine.

12. Bake for about 30 minutes.

Nutritional Information (Per Serving)

Calories: 192

Fat: 1.5g

Sat Fat: 0.2g

Carbohydrates: 34.5g

Fiber: 12g

Sugar: 3.9g

Protein: 11.3g

Sodium: 225mg

Chapter 10: DASH Diet Dessert Recipes

Frozen Fruity Treat

Yield: 6 servings
Preparation Time: 45 minutes
Total Time: 45 minutes
Ingredients:
14-ounce unsweetened almond milk
1 cup frozen pineapple chunks, thawed
4 cups frozen banana slices, thawed
2 tablespoons fresh lime juice
Pinch of salt

Directions:
1. Line glass baking dish with plastic wrap.
2. In high speed blender, add all ingredients and pulse until smooth.
3. Transfer mixture to prepared baking dish and spread evenly.
4. Freeze for about 35-40 minutes before serving.

Nutritional Information (Per Serving)
Calories: 135
Fat: 1.3g
Sat Fat: 0.2g
Carbohydrates: 32.5g
Fiber: 3.3g
Sugar: 20.9g
Protein: 1.5g
Sodium: 77mg

Ricotta Mousse

Yield: 2 servings
Preparation Time: 15 minutes
Total Time: 15 minutes
Ingredients:
2½ cups water, divided
1 cup ricotta cheese
2 teaspoons stevia powder
2 teaspoons cocoa powder
½ teaspoon pure vanilla extract
2 tablespoons fresh blackberries

Directions:
1. In large bowl, add all ingredients except for blackberries and beat until well combined.

2. Transfer mousse into 2 serving glasses and refrigerate to chill for about 4-6 hours or until completely set.

3. Garnish with blackberries and serve.

Nutritional Information (Per Serving)
Calories: 182
Fat: 10.2g
Sat Fat: 6.3g
Carbohydrates: 8.2g
Fiber: 1g
Sugar: 1g
Protein: 14.6g
Sodium: 155mg

Chickpea Fudge

Yield: 12 servings
Preparation Time: 20 minutes
Total Time: 20 minutes
Ingredients:
2 cups chickpeas, cooked
8 Medjool dates, pitted and chopped
½ cup almond butter
½ cup unsweetened almond milk
1 teaspoon vanilla extract
2 tablespoons cocoa powder

Directions:
1. Line a large baking dish with parchment paper.
2. In food processor, add all ingredients except for cocoa powder and pulse until well combined.
3. Transfer mixture to large bowl.
4. Stir in cocoa powder.
5. Divide mixture evenly and transfer to prepared baking dish. Smooth surface with a spatula.
6. Refrigerate for about 2 hours or until completely set.
7. Cut into desired sized squares and serve.

Nutritional Information (Per Serving)
Calories: 146
Fat: 2.7g
Sat Fat: 0.4g
Carbohydrates: 25g
Fiber: 6.6g
Sugar: 7.1g
Protein: 6.9g
Sodium: 16mg

Apple Crisp

Yield: 4 servings
Preparation Time: 15 minutes
Cooking Time: 20 minutes
Total Time: 35 minutes
Ingredients:
For Filling:
2 large Granny Smith apples, peeled, cored, and chopped
2 tablespoons water
2 tablespoons fresh apple juice
¼ teaspoon ground cinnamon

For Topping:
½ cup quick rolled oats
¼ cup unsweetened coconut flakes
2 tablespoons pecans, chopped
½ teaspoon ground cinnamon
¼ cup water

Directions:
1. Preheat oven to 300 degrees F. Lightly grease baking dish.
2. In large mixing bowl, place all filling ingredients and mix gently.
3. Transfer mixture to prepared baking dish.
4. In another bowl, mix together all topping ingredients.
5. Evenly spread topping over filling mixture.
6. Bake for about 20 minutes or until topping is golden brown.

Nutritional Information (Per Serving)
Calories: 194
Fat: 4.1g
Sat Fat: 1.6g

Carbohydrates: 39.5g
Fiber: 23.8g
Sugar: 2.5g
Protein: 6.9g
Sodium: 9mg

Conclusion

High blood pressure is a silent killer that effects millions of people each year. By now you've probably realized that a healthy lifestyle and the DASH diet can help you naturally lower blood pressure. I hope this book helps you take control of your health.

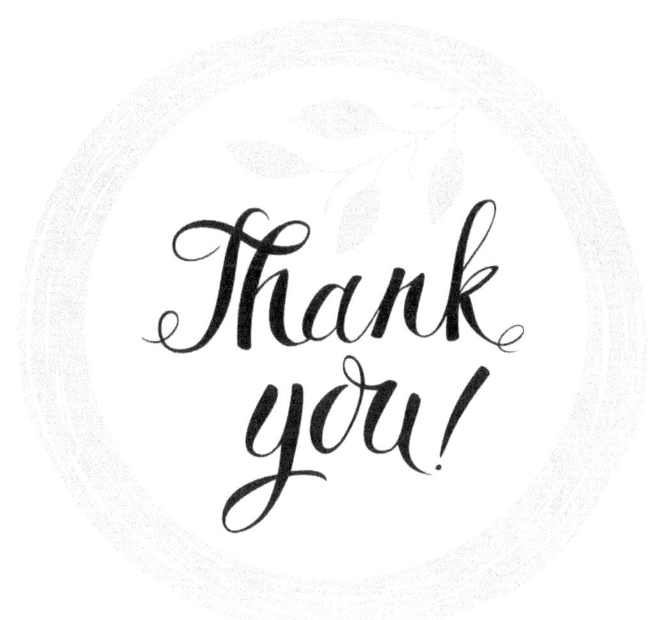

Finally, I want to thank you for reading my book. If you enjoyed the book, please take the time to share your thoughts and post a review on the book retailer's website. It would be greatly appreciated!

Best wishes,

Christina Neal